Bone Health Diet: A Comprehensive Guide To Nourishing Your Bones

By

DR. John Meyers

DR. John Meyers

569 Lexington Ave, New York,

NY 10022

BONE HEALTH DIET

This Book is Dedicated to my beloved wife and child,

Your unwavering love and support have been my rock through every chapter of life. This book is dedicated to you, my pillars of strength and inspiration.

To everyone facing the challenges of a bone-related disorder,

Your resilience and courage in the face of adversity are a testament to the human spirit. May this book serve as a source of knowledge and hope on your journey toward healing and strength.

With love and solidarity,

DR. Meyers.

TABLE OF CONTENTS

Chapter 1: Understanding

Bone Health

Introduction to Bone Health

Strong bones are crucial for overall well-being, providing the structural framework for the body, protecting vital organs, and supporting mobility. In this chapter, we explore the significance of maintaining healthy bones throughout life, understanding their role beyond mere structural support, and how their health impacts our daily lives. We delve into the intricate relationship between bones, diet, and lifestyle, laying the foundation for a comprehensive understanding of bone health.

Anatomy of Bones: Structure and function of bones in the human body.

1. Bone Composition: Bones are complex structures composed of various components, each contributing to their strength and flexibility. The primary components of bones include minerals (such as calcium, phosphorus, and magnesium), collagen (a protein that provides a framework for bone structure), and specialized bone cells (osteoblasts, osteocytes, and osteoclasts) responsible for bone formation, maintenance, and remodeling.

2. Bone Development and Growth: Bone development begins before birth and continues throughout

childhood and adolescence. During growth, bones lengthen and increase in density, primarily due to the process of bone mineralization, where minerals are deposited in the bone matrix, making them stronger. Proper nutrition, especially adequate calcium and vitamin D intake, is crucial during these stages to support optimal bone growth and development.

3. Bone Remodeling: Bone remodeling is a continuous process that occurs throughout life, involving the removal of old bone tissue (resorption) by osteoclasts and the formation of new bone tissue (ossification) by osteoblasts. This process helps maintain bone strength, repair micro-damage, and adapt bones to mechanical stress. Hormonal factors, physical activity, and nutritional factors influence bone remodeling.

4. Bone Density and Strength: Bone density refers to the amount of mineral content in bone tissue, reflecting its strength and resistance to fracture. Peak bone density is typically reached by early adulthood and is influenced by genetics, nutrition, physical activity, and hormonal factors. Low bone density (osteopenia) and significantly reduced bone density

(osteoporosis) increase the risk of fractures and other bone-related issues.

5. Bone Function: Beyond providing structural support for the body, bones serve several essential functions. They act as a reservoir for minerals such as calcium and phosphorus, which are critical for various physiological processes. Additionally, bones house the bone marrow, where hematopoiesis occurs, producing red blood cells, white blood cells, and platelets essential for the body's immune function and oxygen transport. Bones also play a role in regulating mineral homeostasis and acid-base balance in the body.

Common Bone Disorders: Overview of Osteoporosis, Osteopenia, Paget's Disease, and Other Bone-Related Conditions

1. Osteoporosis:
   - Description: Osteoporosis is a condition characterized by a decrease in bone mass and density, leading to increased bone fragility and susceptibility to fractures.
   - Causes: It often occurs due to an imbalance between bone formation and resorption, resulting in weakened bones.
   - Risk Factors: Factors such as aging, female gender, low body weight, hormonal changes, and certain medications can increase the risk of osteoporosis.

- Effects: Osteoporosis can lead to fractures, particularly in the hip, spine, and wrist, which can significantly impact an individual's quality of life.

2. Osteopenia:
   - Description: Osteopenia refers to bone mineral density that is lower than normal but not low enough to be classified as osteoporosis.
   - Causes: Similar to osteoporosis, osteopenia is often caused by an imbalance in bone remodeling processes.
   - Risk Factors: Osteopenia shares many risk factors with osteoporosis, including aging and hormonal changes.
   - Effects: While not as severe as osteoporosis, osteopenia still increases the risk of fractures and can progress to osteoporosis if not managed.

3. Paget's Disease:
   - Description: Paget's disease of bone is a chronic condition characterized by abnormal bone remodeling, leading to enlarged and weakened bones.

BONE HEALTH DIET

  - Causes: The exact cause is not fully understood, but it is believed to involve a combination of genetic and environmental factors.

  - Symptoms: Paget's disease can be asymptomatic or present with bone pain, deformities, fractures, and other complications.

  - Treatment: Treatment aims to reduce symptoms, prevent complications, and maintain bone health through medication and, in some cases, surgery.

4. Other Bone-Related Conditions:

  - Overview: This category includes a range of other bone disorders such as osteomalacia, rickets, bone tumors, and metabolic bone diseases.

  - Causes and Effects: Each condition has its own unique causes, symptoms, and effects on bone health, requiring specific approaches to diagnosis and treatment.

Impact of Diet on Bone Health: How Nutrition Influences Bone Density and Strength

Nutrition plays a crucial role in maintaining optimal bone health throughout life. The foods we consume provide the building blocks necessary for bone formation, maintenance, and repair. Several key nutrients, including calcium, vitamin D, magnesium, vitamin K, and phosphorus, are essential for bone health.

1. Calcium: Calcium is the primary mineral found in bones, providing strength and structure. Adequate calcium intake is vital for bone development in childhood and adolescence and helps prevent bone loss in later years. Dairy products, leafy green vegetables, fortified foods, and certain fish are excellent sources of calcium.

2. Vitamin D: Vitamin D is essential for calcium absorption in the intestines and plays a crucial role in bone mineralization. Sunlight exposure triggers vitamin D synthesis in the skin, while dietary sources include fatty fish, egg yolks, and fortified foods like milk and cereal.

3. Magnesium: Magnesium is involved in bone mineralization and influences bone matrix formation. It works in conjunction with calcium and vitamin D to

support bone health. Nuts, seeds, whole grains, and leafy green vegetables are good sources of magnesium.

4. Vitamin K: Vitamin K is necessary for the activation of proteins involved in bone mineralization. It helps regulate calcium in the bones and blood vessels. Green leafy vegetables, broccoli, and fermented dairy products are rich in vitamin K.

5. Phosphorus: Phosphorus is another mineral that contributes to bone structure, working alongside calcium. It is abundant in protein-rich foods like meat, poultry, fish, dairy products, nuts, and seeds.

In addition to these specific nutrients, a balanced diet that includes adequate protein, fruits, vegetables, and whole grains provides essential vitamins and minerals for overall bone health. Conversely, diets high in sodium, caffeine, and excessive alcohol intake can negatively impact bone health by promoting calcium loss or interfering with nutrient absorption.

BONE HEALTH DIET

Beyond individual nutrients, overall dietary patterns and lifestyle factors also influence bone health. A diet rich in whole foods, including fruits, vegetables, lean proteins, and healthy fats, supports overall health and may benefit bone density. Regular physical activity, particularly weight-bearing exercises like walking, running, and resistance training, helps maintain bone density and strength.

BONE HEALTH DIET

Chapter 2: Nutrients for Bone Health; explain everything in details

Calcium: Importance in Bone Formation and Maintenance

Calcium is a crucial mineral that plays a central role in bone formation, development, and maintenance throughout life. It is the most abundant mineral in the body, with about 99% of the body's calcium stored in the bones and teeth. Calcium is essential for several physiological functions beyond bone health, including muscle contraction, nerve transmission, and blood clotting.

Importance in Bone Formation and Maintenance:

1. Bone Structure: Calcium provides the structural framework for bones, contributing to their strength and density. Adequate calcium intake during childhood and adolescence is critical for building strong bones and reducing the risk of fractures later in life.

2. Bone Remodeling: Throughout life, bones undergo a process called remodeling, where old bone tissue is replaced by new bone tissue. Calcium is necessary for this continuous renewal process, helping to maintain bone strength and integrity.

3. Prevention of Osteoporosis: Insufficient calcium intake over time can lead to a decrease in bone mineral density, increasing the risk of osteoporosis—a condition characterized by weak, brittle bones prone to fractures.

Dietary Sources and Recommended Intake:

1. Food Sources: Calcium is found in a variety of foods, with dairy products such as milk, yogurt, and cheese being the most well-known sources. Other excellent sources of calcium include green leafy vegetables (e.g., kale, broccoli, spinach), fortified plant-based milk alternatives (e.g., almond milk, soy milk), fortified orange juice, canned fish with bones (e.g., sardines, salmon), and certain nuts and seeds (e.g., almonds, sesame seeds).

2. Supplements: In cases where dietary intake alone is insufficient, calcium supplements may be recommended. These supplements should be taken in consultation with a healthcare professional to ensure they are appropriate and safe, as excessive calcium intake can have adverse effects.

Recommended Intake:

The recommended dietary allowance (RDA) for calcium varies by age and gender:
- Adults aged 19-50: 1,000 milligrams (mg) per day
- Women aged 51 and older: 1,200 mg per day
- Men aged 51-70: 1,000 mg per day
- Men aged 71 and older: 1,200 mg per day

It's important to note that the body's ability to absorb calcium depends on several factors, including vitamin D levels, overall diet, and individual differences in absorption. Consuming calcium-rich foods as part of a balanced diet is the most effective way to ensure adequate intake and support optimal bone health.

Vitamin D: Role in Calcium Absorption and Bone Health

Vitamin D is a fat-soluble vitamin that plays a crucial role in calcium absorption and bone health. Its primary function is to regulate calcium and phosphorus levels in the body, essential minerals for bone mineralization and overall skeletal health. Here's a detailed look at the role of vitamin D in bone health and its sources:

1. Calcium Absorption: Vitamin D enhances the absorption of dietary calcium in the intestines. When there is insufficient vitamin D, the body struggles to absorb adequate calcium, leading to weakened bones and an increased risk of fractures. By promoting

calcium absorption, vitamin D helps maintain proper bone density and strength.

2. Bone Mineralization: Vitamin D is involved in the process of bone mineralization, where calcium and phosphorus are deposited into the bone matrix, contributing to bone density and structure. Without sufficient vitamin D, the body cannot effectively utilize the calcium obtained from the diet, leading to weakened bones.

3. Regulation of Calcium and Phosphorus: Vitamin D helps regulate calcium and phosphorus levels in the blood, ensuring a proper balance that is crucial for bone health. This balance is essential for various cellular functions and maintaining the integrity of the skeletal system.

4. Sun Exposure: The primary natural source of vitamin D is sunlight. When the skin is exposed to UVB radiation from the sun, it triggers the production of vitamin D in the skin. The amount of sunlight needed varies based on factors such as skin type, time of day, season, and geographic location. Generally, about 10-

30 minutes of sun exposure to the face, arms, and legs a few times a week is sufficient for most people to produce an adequate amount of vitamin D.

5. Dietary Sources: While sunlight is the primary natural source, vitamin D can also be obtained from certain foods and supplements. Dietary sources of vitamin D include fatty fish (such as salmon, mackerel, and tuna), egg yolks, fortified dairy products (milk, yogurt, cheese), fortified plant-based milk (soy, almond), fortified cereals, and some types of mushrooms.

6. Supplementation: In cases where adequate sun exposure or dietary sources are not available, vitamin D supplements may be recommended. These supplements are available in various forms, including vitamin D2 (ergocalciferol) and vitamin D3 (cholecalciferol), with vitamin D3 being the preferred form for supplementation due to its superior bioavailability.

7. Health Implications: Vitamin D deficiency can lead to a variety of health problems, including weakened

bones (osteomalacia in adults, rickets in children), increased risk of fractures, muscle weakness, and a compromised immune system. Maintaining adequate vitamin D levels is essential for overall health and well-being, especially for bone health.

Appropriate Intake of Vitamin D Across Age Groups:

1. Infants (0-12 months): The American Academy of Pediatrics (AAP) recommends that exclusively breastfed infants receive a vitamin D supplement of 400 IU per day, beginning in the first few days of life. For formula-fed infants, the vitamin D content in formula typically meets their needs.

2. Children (1-18 years): The recommended daily intake of vitamin D for children and adolescents is 600 IU per day. This can be obtained from a combination of sunlight exposure, dietary sources, and supplements if necessary.

3. Adults (19-70 years): The recommended daily intake of vitamin D for adults is 600 IU per day. Older adults

may require higher amounts, especially if they have limited sun exposure or other risk factors for deficiency.

4. Older Adults (71 years and older): The recommended daily intake of vitamin D for older adults is 800 IU per day. As people age, their skin becomes less efficient at producing vitamin D from sunlight, making supplementation or dietary sources more important.

5. Pregnant and Breastfeeding Women: Pregnant and breastfeeding women have higher vitamin D needs. The recommended daily intake is 600 IU per day during pregnancy and lactation.

It's important to note that individual needs may vary based on factors such as skin color, geographic location, sun exposure, dietary habits, and health status. Some individuals may require higher doses of vitamin D to maintain optimal levels, especially if they have limited sun exposure or conditions that affect vitamin D absorption. Consulting with a healthcare provider can help determine the appropriate vitamin

D intake for specific needs. Regular monitoring of vitamin D levels through blood tests may also be recommended to ensure adequacy.

Magnesium: Contribution to Bone Health and Dietary Sources

Magnesium is a vital mineral that plays a critical role in maintaining bone health. It is the fourth most abundant mineral in the human body and is involved in various physiological processes, including bone formation, mineralization, and metabolism. Here's a detailed look at the contribution of magnesium to bone health and its dietary sources:

1. Bone Formation: Magnesium is essential for the activation of vitamin D, which, in turn, is necessary for calcium absorption in the intestines. This process is crucial for the mineralization of newly formed bone tissue. Magnesium also supports the synthesis of bone-building proteins and enzymes, contributing to the overall structure and strength of bones.

2. Regulation of Calcium Levels: Magnesium helps regulate calcium levels within the body by influencing the activity of parathyroid hormone (PTH) and calcitonin. These hormones play a role in maintaining calcium balance in the blood and bones, which is essential for bone health.

3. Bone Density: Studies have suggested that magnesium intake is positively associated with bone mineral density (BMD). Higher BMD is linked to reduced fracture risk and better overall bone health, highlighting the importance of magnesium in maintaining bone density.

4. Dietary Sources: Magnesium is naturally found in a variety of foods, with some of the richest sources including:
   - Nuts and Seeds: Almonds, cashews, peanuts, pumpkin seeds, and sesame seeds are excellent sources of magnesium.
   - Whole Grains: Whole wheat, oats, quinoa, and brown rice contain magnesium, particularly in the germ and bran portions of the grain.

- Legumes: Beans, lentils, chickpeas, and peas are good plant-based sources of magnesium.
- Leafy

Green Vegetables: Spinach, kale, Swiss chard, and other dark leafy greens are rich in magnesium.
- Seafood: Some types of fish, such as mackerel and salmon, are good sources of magnesium.
- Dairy Products: Milk, yogurt, and cheese contain magnesium, with higher concentrations found in the whey portion of milk.

5. Bioavailability: While magnesium is present in many foods, its bioavailability can be affected by factors such as food processing, cooking methods, and the presence of other nutrients. Consuming a varied diet that includes a range of magnesium-rich foods can help ensure adequate intake.

6. Recommended Intake: The Recommended Dietary Allowance (RDA) for magnesium varies by age and gender, with adult males needing around 400-420 mg per day and adult females needing 310-320 mg per

day. Pregnant and lactating women have slightly higher magnesium requirements.

7. Supplementation: In some cases, supplementation may be necessary to meet magnesium needs, especially for individuals with low dietary intake or specific health conditions. However, it's essential to consult with a healthcare professional before starting any supplementation regimen to determine individual needs and potential interactions with other medications or health conditions.

Other Essential Nutrients for Bone Health

In addition to calcium and vitamin D, several other nutrients play critical roles in maintaining optimal bone health. These nutrients contribute to various aspects of bone formation, structure, and mineralization, and their adequate intake is essential for preserving bone density and strength.

1. Vitamin K: Vitamin K is known for its role in blood clotting, but it also plays a crucial role in bone metabolism. There are two main forms of vitamin K:

K1 (phylloquinone), found in green leafy vegetables like spinach and kale, and K2 (menaquinone), found in fermented foods and animal products. Vitamin K activates proteins involved in bone mineralization, helping to bind calcium to the bone matrix and prevent its accumulation in soft tissues.

2. Phosphorus: Phosphorus is a mineral that works closely with calcium to form the structural component of bone mineral. It is the second most abundant mineral in the body, found in high amounts in dairy products, meat, fish, poultry, and whole grains. Phosphorus is essential for maintaining the strength and integrity of bones and teeth, and it plays a critical role in the body's energy production and storage.

3. Trace Minerals: Trace minerals, including zinc, copper, manganese, and boron, are essential for bone health in small amounts. These minerals are involved in various biochemical processes related to bone metabolism, such as collagen synthesis, antioxidant defense, and enzymatic reactions. While they are required in smaller quantities compared to major

minerals like calcium and phosphorus, their roles in bone health should not be overlooked.

- Zinc: Zinc is involved in bone mineralization and collagen synthesis. It supports the activity of osteoblasts, the cells responsible for bone formation. Dietary sources of zinc include meat, shellfish, legumes, seeds, and nuts.

- Copper: Copper is required for the cross-linking of collagen fibers in bone tissue, contributing to bone strength and flexibility. Foods rich in copper include organ meats, shellfish, nuts, seeds, and whole grains.

- Manganese: Manganese plays a role in bone mineralization and the formation of connective tissue. It is found in nuts, seeds, whole grains, legumes, and leafy green vegetables.

- Boron: Boron is involved in the metabolism of calcium, magnesium, and phosphorus, influencing bone mineral density and strength. It is found in fruits, vegetables, nuts, and legumes.

BONE HEALTH DIET

Bone Health Diet

Chapter 3: Diet for Osteoporosis Prevention and Management

Understanding Osteoporosis: Risk Factors, Prevention Strategies, and Treatment Options

Osteoporosis is a condition characterized by weakened bones that are more susceptible to fractures. It is often referred to as a "silent disease" because it progresses without noticeable symptoms until a fracture occurs. Understanding the risk factors, prevention strategies, and treatment options for osteoporosis is crucial for managing and reducing the risk of this condition.

1. Risk Factors: Several factors can increase the risk of developing osteoporosis, including:

  - Age: The risk of osteoporosis increases with age, particularly in postmenopausal women due to hormonal changes.
  - Gender: Women are more prone to osteoporosis than men, especially after menopause.
  - Family History: A family history of osteoporosis or fractures can increase the risk.
  - Low Body Weight: Having a low body weight or a small frame can increase the risk of osteoporosis.
  - Hormonal Changes: Reduced estrogen levels in women and low testosterone levels in men can contribute to bone loss.

Bone Health Diet

- Nutrition: Poor nutrition, particularly low calcium and vitamin D intake, can weaken bones.
- Sedentary Lifestyle: Lack of physical activity and weight-bearing exercises can lead to bone loss.
- Smoking and Alcohol: Smoking and excessive alcohol consumption can negatively impact bone health.

2. Prevention Strategies: Prevention of osteoporosis involves lifestyle modifications and dietary changes to support bone health:

- Adequate Calcium and Vitamin D: Ensure sufficient intake of calcium-rich foods and vitamin D to support bone strength.
- Regular Exercise: Engage in weight-bearing and muscle-strengthening exercises to promote bone density.
- Healthy Lifestyle: Avoid smoking, limit alcohol consumption, and maintain a healthy body weight.
- Fall Prevention: Take measures to prevent falls, such as improving home safety and using assistive devices if needed.

BONE HEALTH DIET

3. Treatment Options: Treatment for osteoporosis aims to prevent fractures and maintain bone strength:

- Medications: Various medications, including bisphosphonates, hormone therapy, and bone-building medications, may be prescribed to prevent bone loss or increase bone density.
- Lifestyle Changes: Dietary modifications, exercise programs, and lifestyle adjustments can complement medical treatment.
- Fall Prevention: Implementing strategies to prevent falls, such as improving balance and strength through exercise, can reduce the risk of fractures.

Calcium-Rich Foods: Incorporating Dairy and Non-Dairy Sources of Calcium into the Diet

Calcium is a key nutrient for building and maintaining strong bones. It is essential for bone health, and getting an adequate amount of calcium through diet is crucial for preventing osteoporosis and maintaining bone density. Both dairy and non-dairy sources of calcium can be included in the diet to meet daily calcium needs.

1. Dairy Sources of Calcium:

 - Milk: Cow's milk is a rich source of calcium. It can be consumed as a beverage or used in cooking and baking.

 - Yogurt: Yogurt is another dairy product that is high in calcium. Opt for plain yogurt without added sugars for a healthier option.

 - Cheese: Cheese, such as cheddar, mozzarella, and Swiss, provides a good amount of calcium. However, it's important to consume cheese in moderation due to its high fat and calorie content.

2. Non-Dairy Sources of Calcium:

 - Leafy Greens: Dark leafy greens like kale, collard greens, turnip greens, and bok choy are excellent sources of calcium. They can be incorporated into salads, soups, stir-fries, or smoothies.

 - Fortified Foods: Many non-dairy milk alternatives, such as almond milk, soy milk, and oat milk, are fortified with calcium and other nutrients. Look for products labeled as "fortified" to ensure adequate calcium intake.

- Tofu: Tofu, made from soybeans, is a plant-based source of calcium. It can be used in various dishes, including stir-fries, salads, and smoothies.

- Nuts and Seeds: Some nuts and seeds, such as almonds, sesame seeds, and chia seeds, contain calcium. They can be enjoyed as snacks or added to meals for a calcium boost.

3. Tips for Incorporating Calcium-Rich Foods:

- Include a variety of calcium sources in your diet to ensure you're getting enough of this essential nutrient.

- Aim to include at least three servings of calcium-rich foods in your daily meals and snacks.

- Read food labels to check the calcium content of packaged foods and choose products with higher calcium levels.

- Consider using calcium-fortified foods and beverages as convenient sources of calcium, especially if you have dietary restrictions or preferences that limit dairy consumption.

Vitamin D Supplementation: Guidelines for Vitamin D Intake and Supplements

Vitamin D is essential for calcium absorption and bone health. While sunlight exposure triggers the body's natural production of vitamin D, many people may not get enough sunlight or dietary sources of vitamin D to meet their needs, especially in regions with limited sunlight or during certain seasons. Therefore, supplementation with vitamin D may be necessary to maintain optimal levels, particularly for individuals at risk of or with osteoporosis.

1. Recommended Intake: The recommended dietary allowance (RDA) for vitamin D varies based on age, sex, and other factors. For adults up to age 70, the RDA is 600 international units (IU) per day, while adults over 70 should aim for 800 IU per day. However, individual requirements may vary, and some experts suggest higher doses for certain populations, such as those with limited sun exposure or specific health conditions.

2. Sources of Vitamin D: In addition to sunlight exposure, dietary sources of vitamin D include fatty fish (e.g., salmon, mackerel, tuna), egg yolks, fortified

dairy products (e.g., milk, yogurt, cheese), fortified plant-based milk alternatives, and some fortified cereals and juices. However, it can be challenging to obtain adequate vitamin D from diet alone, especially for those with limited dietary sources or absorption issues.

3. Supplementation Guidelines: For individuals at risk of vitamin D deficiency or those with osteoporosis, supplementation may be recommended to achieve and maintain optimal vitamin D levels. Vitamin D supplements are available in various forms, including vitamin D2 (ergocalciferol) and vitamin D3 (cholecalciferol). Vitamin D3 is the preferred form, as it is more effective at raising and maintaining vitamin D levels in the body.

4. Consultation with Healthcare Provider: Before starting vitamin D supplementation, it is important to consult with a healthcare provider to determine the appropriate dosage based on individual needs and to monitor vitamin D levels over time. Blood tests can assess vitamin D status and guide supplementation decisions.

5. Combination with Calcium: Vitamin D works synergistically with calcium in bone health. Therefore, for individuals at risk of or with osteoporosis, combining vitamin D supplementation with adequate calcium intake is often recommended to support bone density and reduce the risk of fractures.

6. Sunlight Exposure: While vitamin D supplements can help maintain adequate levels, safe exposure to sunlight remains an important natural source of vitamin D synthesis. Spending time outdoors, especially during midday when the sun is strongest, can help the body produce vitamin D. However, it is important to balance sunlight exposure to minimize the risk of skin damage from UV radiation.

Anti-Inflammatory Diet for Osteoporosis Prevention and Management

An anti-inflammatory diet focuses on consuming foods that have been shown to reduce inflammation in the body. Chronic inflammation can contribute to bone loss and osteoporosis, so adopting an anti-inflammatory eating pattern may help support bone health. The following are key components of an anti-inflammatory diet that may benefit individuals at risk of or managing osteoporosis:

1. Fruits and Vegetables: Colorful fruits and vegetables are rich in antioxidants and phytochemicals that can help reduce inflammation. Aim to include a variety of fruits and vegetables in your diet, such as berries, leafy greens, tomatoes, bell peppers, and cruciferous vegetables like broccoli and Brussels sprouts.

2. Healthy Fats: Certain fats, particularly omega-3 fatty acids found in fatty fish (e.g., salmon, mackerel, sardines), flaxseeds, chia seeds, and walnuts, have anti-inflammatory properties. Additionally, monounsaturated fats found in olive oil, avocados, and nuts can help reduce inflammation.

3. Whole Grains: Whole grains like brown rice, quinoa, oats, and whole wheat contain fiber and nutrients that may have anti-inflammatory effects. Avoid refined grains and products made with white flour, as these can contribute to inflammation.

BONE HEALTH DIET

4. Lean Proteins: Include lean sources of protein in your diet, such as poultry, fish, legumes, and tofu. These foods provide essential amino acids for bone health without the added saturated fat found in some animal proteins.

5. Herbs and Spices: Certain herbs and spices, such as turmeric, ginger, garlic, and cinnamon, have been shown to possess anti-inflammatory properties. Incorporate these flavorful ingredients into your meals to boost their anti-inflammatory potential.

6. Dairy or Dairy Alternatives: Calcium and vitamin D are crucial for bone health, so it's important to include dairy products or fortified alternatives in your diet. Opt for low-fat or non-fat dairy options to minimize saturated fat intake.

7. Limit Sugar and Processed Foods: High-sugar foods and processed foods can contribute to inflammation. Limit your intake of sugary snacks, sodas, and processed snacks to reduce inflammation and support overall health.

Bone Health Diet

8. Hydration: Staying hydrated is essential for overall health, including bone health. Aim to drink plenty of water throughout the day to support proper hydration.

Chapter 4: Bone-Friendly

Recipes

Bone-Friendly Breakfast Ideas for

Optimal Bone Health

Starting your day with a nutritious breakfast is essential for maintaining energy levels and supporting overall health, including bone health. Here are some bone-friendly breakfast ideas that incorporate key nutrients for optimal bone health:

1. Greek Yogurt Parfait:
  - Ingredients:

- *Greek yogurt (plain or flavored)*
- *Mixed berries (e.g., strawberries, blueberries, raspberries)*
- *Granola or chopped nuts*
- *Honey or maple syrup (optional)*
- *Instructions:*
- *In a bowl or glass, layer Greek yogurt with mixed berries and granola or chopped nuts.*
- *Drizzle with honey or maple syrup for added sweetness if desired.*

2. Spinach and Feta Omelet:
  - *Ingredients:*
    - *Eggs*
    - *Fresh spinach leaves*
    - *Feta cheese (crumbled)*
    - *Olive oil*
    - *Salt and pepper to taste*
  - *Instructions:*
    - *In a bowl, beat eggs with salt and pepper.*
    - *In a non-stick skillet, heat olive oil over medium heat. Add fresh spinach leaves and cook until wilted.*

- Pour the beaten eggs over the spinach and cook until set. Sprinkle crumbled feta cheese on top.

- Fold the omelet in half and cook for an additional minute or until the cheese melts.

3. Oatmeal with Chia Seeds and Almonds:
  - Ingredients:
    - Rolled oats
    - Chia seeds
    - Almonds (chopped)
    - Milk (dairy or plant-based)
    - Honey or maple syrup (optional)
  - Instructions:
    - Cook rolled oats according to package instructions, using milk instead of water for added calcium.
    - Stir in chia seeds and chopped almonds.
    - Sweeten with honey or maple syrup if desired.

4. Whole Grain Pancakes with Berries:
  - Ingredients:
    - Whole grain pancake mix
    - Mixed berries (fresh or frozen)

- *Greek yogurt (optional)*
- *Instructions:*
- *Prepare whole grain pancake batter according to package instructions.*
- *Cook pancakes on a griddle or skillet until golden brown.*
- *Serve with mixed berries on top and a dollop of Greek yogurt if desired.*

5. *Smoothie Bowl:*
  - *Ingredients:*
    - *Frozen mixed berries*
    - *Banana*
    - *Spinach or kale leaves*
    - *Greek yogurt or milk (dairy or plant-based)*
    - *Toppings: granola, nuts, seeds, shredded coconut*
  - *Instructions:*
    - *Blend frozen berries, banana, spinach or kale, and Greek yogurt or milk until smooth.*
    - *Pour the smoothie into a bowl and add toppings like granola, nuts, seeds, or shredded coconut for added texture and nutrients.*

Lunch and Dinner Recipes for Bone Health

Incorporating bone-healthy ingredients into your meals can be both nutritious and delicious. Here are some lunch and dinner recipes that feature ingredients known for their benefits to bone health:

1. Salmon and Quinoa Salad:
  - Ingredients:
    - Grilled salmon fillet
    - Cooked quinoa
    - Mixed greens (spinach, kale, arugula)
    - Cherry tomatoes
    - Cucumber slices
    - Avocado slices
    - Lemon vinaigrette (olive oil, lemon juice, Dijon mustard, salt, and pepper)

  - Directions:
    - In a large bowl, combine the mixed greens, quinoa, cherry tomatoes, and cucumber slices.
    - Top the salad with grilled salmon and avocado slices.

- Drizzle the lemon vinaigrette over the salad and toss gently to combine.

2. Vegetable Stir-Fry with Tofu:
  - Ingredients:
    - Firm tofu, cubed
    - Assorted vegetables (bell peppers, broccoli, snap peas, carrots)
    - Garlic and ginger, minced
    - Low-sodium soy sauce
    - Sesame oil
    - Brown rice or quinoa (optional)

  - Directions:
    - In a large skillet or wok, heat sesame oil over medium-high heat.
    - Add the tofu cubes and stir-fry until golden brown.
    - Add the minced garlic and ginger, followed by the assorted vegetables.
    - Stir-fry the vegetables until tender-crisp.
    - Add a splash of low-sodium soy sauce and toss to combine.

- Serve the stir-fry over brown rice or quinoa if desired.

3. Mediterranean Chicken Skewers:
  - Ingredients:
    - Chicken breast, cut into cubes
    - Cherry tomatoes
    - Red onion, cut into chunks
    - Bell peppers, cut into chunks
    - Olive oil
    - Lemon juice
    - Fresh herbs (rosemary, thyme, oregano)
    - Salt and pepper

  - Directions:
    - Preheat the grill to medium-high heat.
    - Thread the chicken cubes, cherry tomatoes, red onion, and bell peppers onto skewers.
    - In a small bowl, whisk together olive oil, lemon juice, fresh herbs, salt, and pepper to make a marinade.
    - Brush the marinade over the skewers.

- Grill the skewers for 10-12 minutes, turning occasionally, until the chicken is cooked through and the vegetables are charred.

4. Spinach and Feta Stuffed Chicken Breast:
  - Ingredients:
    - Boneless, skinless chicken breasts
    - Fresh spinach leaves
    - Feta cheese
    - Garlic, minced
    - Olive oil
    - Salt and pepper

  - Directions:
    - Preheat the oven to 375°F (190°C).
    - Flatten the chicken breasts and season with salt and pepper.
    - In a skillet, sauté the spinach and garlic in olive oil until wilted.
    - Remove from heat and stir in crumbled feta cheese.
    - Spoon the spinach and feta mixture onto each chicken breast.

- *Roll up the chicken breasts and secure with toothpicks.*

- *Place the chicken rolls in a baking dish and bake for 25-30 minutes or until the chicken is cooked through.*

5. *Bean and Vegetable Chili:*
   - *Ingredients:*
   - *Mixed beans (kidney beans, black beans, pinto beans)*
   - *Diced tomatoes*
   - *Bell peppers, diced*
   - *Onion, diced*
   - *Garlic, minced*
   - *Chili powder, cumin, paprika*
   - *Vegetable broth*
   - *Olive oil*
   - *Salt and pepper*

   - *Directions:*
   - *In a large pot, heat olive oil over medium heat.*
   - *Add the diced onions, bell peppers, and garlic, and sauté until softened.*

- Stir in the mixed beans, diced tomatoes, chili powder, cumin, paprika, and vegetable broth.
- Bring the chili to a simmer and cook for 20-25 minutes, stirring occasionally.
- Season with salt and pepper to taste.

6. Grilled Vegetable and Quinoa Salad:
   - Ingredients:
     - Quinoa, cooked
     - Assorted vegetables (zucchini, eggplant, bell peppers)
     - Cherry tomatoes
     - Red onion, thinly sliced
     - Balsamic vinaigrette
     - Fresh basil leaves
     - Olive oil
     - Salt and pepper

   - Directions:
     - Preheat the grill to medium-high heat.
     - Brush the vegetables with olive oil and season with salt and pepper.
     - Grill the vegetables until tender and slightly charred.

- In a large bowl, combine the cooked quinoa, grilled vegetables, cherry tomatoes, and red onion.
- Drizzle with balsamic vinaigrette and toss gently to combine.
- Garnish with fresh basil leaves before serving.

7. Lentil and Vegetable Curry:
  - Ingredients:
    - Lentils, cooked
    - Mixed vegetables (carrots, peas, cauliflower)
    - Onion, diced
    - Garlic, minced
    - Ginger, grated
    - Curry powder, turmeric, cumin
    - Coconut milk
    - Vegetable broth
    - Olive oil
    - Salt and pepper

  - Directions:
    - In a large pot, heat olive oil over medium heat.
    - Add the diced onions, garlic, and ginger, and sauté until fragrant.

- Stir in the curry powder, turmeric, and cumin, and cook for another minute.

- Add the mixed vegetables, cooked lentils, coconut milk, and vegetable broth.

- Bring the curry to a simmer and cook for 15-20 minutes, or until the vegetables are tender.

- Season with salt and pepper to taste.

8. Turkey and Vegetable Skewers:

- Ingredients:

- Turkey breast, cut into cubes

- Cherry tomatoes

- Mushrooms, halved

- Red onion, cut into chunks

- Zucchini, sliced

- Olive oil

- Lemon juice

- Fresh herbs (rosemary, thyme, oregano)

- Salt and pepper

- Directions:

- Preheat the grill to medium-high heat.

- Thread the turkey cubes, cherry tomatoes, mushrooms, red onion, and zucchini onto skewers.

- In a small bowl, whisk together olive oil, lemon juice, fresh herbs, salt, and pepper to make a marinade.

- Brush the marinade over the skewers.

- Grill the skewers for 10-12 minutes, turning occasionally, until the turkey is cooked through and the vegetables are tender.

Snacks and Desserts: Healthy Options for Bone Health

Snacking and enjoying desserts can be a part of a bone-healthy diet when you choose nutrient-dense options that provide essential vitamins and minerals. Here are some delicious and nutritious snack and dessert ideas that can support bone health:

1. Cottage Cheese with Fruit: Top cottage cheese with your choice of fresh or dried fruits, such as berries, peaches, or apricots, for a protein-rich snack that's also high in calcium. Simply spoon cottage cheese into a bowl and add your favorite fruits.

2. Hummus and Veggie Sticks: Serve hummus with a variety of colorful vegetable sticks, such as carrots, bell peppers, and cucumber slices, for a fiber-rich snack that provides vitamins and minerals. Simply chop the vegetables into sticks and serve alongside hummus.

3. Apple Slices with Almond Butter: Spread almond butter on apple slices for a crunchy and satisfying snack that's rich in calcium, magnesium, and healthy fats. Simply slice an apple and spread almond butter on each slice.

4. Greek Yogurt with Honey and Nuts: Mix Greek yogurt with a drizzle of honey and a sprinkle of nuts, such as almonds or walnuts, for a creamy and protein-packed snack that's high in calcium. Simply spoon Greek yogurt into a bowl, add honey and nuts, and mix well.

5. Whole Grain Crackers with Cheese: Pair whole grain crackers with your favorite cheese for a calcium-rich snack that also provides fiber and protein. Simply place cheese slices on top of whole grain crackers.

BONE HEALTH DIET

6. Popcorn with Nutritional Yeast: Sprinkle air-popped popcorn with nutritional yeast for a savory and crunchy snack that's rich in B vitamins and minerals like magnesium. Simply pop the popcorn and sprinkle with nutritional yeast.

7. Cherry Tomato and Mozzarella Skewers: Thread cherry tomatoes and small mozzarella balls onto skewers for a colorful and calcium-rich snack that's also high in vitamin C. Simply skewer the tomatoes and mozzarella balls.

8. Hard-Boiled Eggs: Enjoy hard-boiled eggs as a convenient and protein-rich snack that's also high in nutrients like vitamin D and phosphorus. Simply boil eggs until they're cooked to your desired doneness.

9. Avocado Toast: Spread mashed avocado on whole grain toast for a satisfying and nutrient-dense snack that's rich in healthy fats, fiber, and vitamins like K and C. Simply mash avocado and spread it on toasted bread.

10. Homemade Energy Balls: Combine nuts, seeds, dried fruits, and a touch of honey in a food processor, then roll into bite-sized balls for a convenient and nutrient-packed snack that's high in calcium, magnesium, and fiber. Simply blend the ingredients in a food processor, roll into balls, and refrigerate.

11. Yogurt Parfait: Layer low-fat yogurt with fresh berries and a sprinkle of nuts or seeds for a calcium-rich snack packed with protein and antioxidants.

12. Homemade Trail Mix: Create your own trail mix by combining unsalted nuts (such as almonds, walnuts, or pistachios), seeds (like pumpkin or sunflower seeds), and dried fruits (such as apricots or raisins) for a satisfying snack rich in magnesium and potassium.

13. Smoothie Bowl: Blend together your favorite fruits with yogurt or milk, and top with granola, nuts, or seeds for a refreshing and calcium-packed snack or dessert.

14. Dark Chocolate-Covered Almonds: Dip almonds in melted dark chocolate and let them cool for a

BONE HEALTH DIET

crunchy, indulgent treat that provides a dose of calcium, magnesium, and antioxidants.

15. Baked Fruit: Roast apples, pears, or peaches with a sprinkle of cinnamon and a drizzle of honey for a warm, naturally sweet dessert that's high in fiber and vitamin C.

16. Chia Seed Pudding: Mix chia seeds with milk or a dairy-free alternative, sweeten with a touch of honey or maple syrup, and let it set in the refrigerator for a creamy, calcium-rich pudding.

17. Greek Yogurt Bark: Spread Greek yogurt on a baking sheet, top with fruits, nuts, and a drizzle of honey, and freeze until firm. Break into pieces for a satisfying and calcium-packed snack.

18. Frozen Banana Bites: Dip banana slices in yogurt or nut butter, then roll in crushed nuts or seeds. Freeze until firm for a creamy, crunchy snack that's rich in potassium and calcium.

Chapter 5: Diet for Arthritis

and Joint Health

Types of Arthritis: Overview of Osteoarthritis, Rheumatoid Arthritis, and Other Joint Conditions

Arthritis encompasses a range of conditions that affect the joints, causing pain, stiffness, and reduced mobility. Understanding the different types of arthritis is crucial for implementing dietary strategies that can help manage symptoms and support joint health. Here are the key types of arthritis and their characteristics:

1. Osteoarthritis (OA): Osteoarthritis is the most common form of arthritis, characterized by the breakdown of cartilage in the joints. It typically occurs in weight-bearing joints such as the knees, hips, and spine, as well as in the hands. OA is often associated with aging, joint injury, and obesity. Symptoms include joint pain, stiffness, and reduced range of motion.

2. Rheumatoid Arthritis (RA): Rheumatoid arthritis is an autoimmune disease that causes chronic inflammation of the joints. It can affect multiple joints throughout the body, leading to pain, swelling, and joint deformity. RA is caused by the immune system mistakenly attacking the synovium (the lining of the membranes that surround the joints). It is characterized by periods of flare-ups and remission.

3. Other Joint Conditions: In addition to OA and RA, there are other types of arthritis and joint conditions that can impact joint health. These may include gout, lupus-related arthritis, psoriatic arthritis, ankylosing spondylitis, and others. Each of these conditions has its own unique characteristics and may require specific dietary considerations for management.

Managing Arthritis and Joint Health through Diet:

- Anti-Inflammatory Diet: Many individuals with arthritis find relief from symptoms by following an anti-inflammatory diet. This diet focuses on consuming foods that reduce inflammation in the body, such as fruits, vegetables, whole grains, healthy fats (like those found in fish and nuts), and spices like turmeric and ginger.

- Omega-3 Fatty Acids: Omega-3 fatty acids, found in fatty fish (such as salmon, mackerel, and sardines), flaxseeds, chia seeds, and walnuts, have anti-inflammatory properties that can help reduce joint pain and stiffness.

- Calcium and Vitamin D: Adequate intake of calcium and vitamin D is important for maintaining bone density and overall joint health. Dairy products, fortified plant-based milks, leafy green vegetables, and exposure to sunlight are good sources of these nutrients.

- Weight Management: For individuals with arthritis, maintaining a healthy weight is essential, as excess weight can put added stress on the joints. A balanced diet that supports weight management can help reduce joint pain and improve mobility.

Incorporating Anti-Inflammatory Foods for Arthritis and Joint Health

A diet rich in anti-inflammatory foods can help manage inflammation and reduce joint pain associated with arthritis. By including these foods in your daily meals, you can support joint health and potentially alleviate symptoms. Here are some key anti-inflammatory foods to incorporate into your diet:

1. Fatty Fish: Fatty fish such as salmon, mackerel, sardines, and trout are rich in omega-3 fatty acids, which have been shown to reduce inflammation. Aim to include fatty fish in your diet several times a week.

2. Berries: Berries like strawberries, blueberries, raspberries, and blackberries are high in antioxidants called polyphenols, which can help reduce inflammation. Add a handful of berries to your breakfast or snack on them throughout the day.

3. Leafy Greens: Dark, leafy greens like spinach, kale, and Swiss chard are packed with vitamins, minerals, and antioxidants that can help fight inflammation. Include a variety of leafy greens in salads, smoothies, or cooked dishes.

4. Nuts and Seeds: Nuts and seeds, such as almonds, walnuts, flaxseeds, and chia seeds, are rich in omega-3 fatty acids and other anti-inflammatory compounds. Snack on a handful of nuts or sprinkle seeds on salads and yogurt.

BONE HEALTH DIET

5. Turmeric: Turmeric contains a compound called curcumin, which has powerful anti-inflammatory properties. Add turmeric to curries, soups, or smoothies for its potential health benefits.

6. Ginger: Ginger is another spice known for its anti-inflammatory effects. Use fresh ginger in cooking, or brew ginger tea to enjoy its soothing properties.

7. Extra Virgin Olive Oil: Extra virgin olive oil is rich in monounsaturated fats and contains anti-inflammatory compounds. Use it for salad dressings or drizzle it over cooked vegetables.

8. Garlic: Garlic contains sulfur compounds that have been shown to have anti-inflammatory effects. Add fresh garlic to your meals for a flavorful and healthful boost.

9. Green Tea: Green tea is high in antioxidants known as catechins, which have anti-inflammatory effects. Enjoy a cup of green tea as a refreshing beverage.

10. Whole Grains: Whole grains like brown rice, quinoa, barley, and oats contain fiber and nutrients that can help reduce inflammation. Replace refined grains with whole grains for added health benefits.

Omega-3 Fatty Acids for Arthritis and Joint Health

Omega-3 fatty acids are essential fats with anti-inflammatory properties that have been linked to various health benefits, including improved joint health and reduced inflammation associated with arthritis. Incorporating omega-3s into your diet may help manage symptoms of arthritis and support overall joint health. Here's what you need to know about omega-3 fatty acids and their sources:

1. Benefits for Joint Health: Omega-3 fatty acids, particularly eicosapentaenoic acid (EPA) and docosahexaenoic acid (DHA), have been shown to reduce inflammation in the body, which can benefit individuals with arthritis by easing joint pain, stiffness, and swelling. Omega-3s may also help slow down the progression of joint damage in certain types of arthritis.

2. Sources of Omega-3s: The primary dietary sources of omega-3 fatty acids are fatty fish, such as salmon, mackerel, sardines, trout, and herring. These fish are rich in EPA and DHA, the most bioavailable forms of omega-3s. Other sources of omega-3s include flaxseeds, chia seeds, hemp seeds, walnuts, and algae-based supplements.

3. Fish Oil Supplements: For individuals who may not consume enough omega-3-rich foods, fish oil supplements can be a convenient way to increase omega-3 intake. Fish oil supplements typically contain concentrated amounts of EPA and DHA, and they are available in liquid, capsule, or softgel form. It's important to choose high-quality supplements from reputable brands to ensure purity and potency.

4. Balancing Omega-3 and Omega-6 Fatty Acids: While omega-3 fatty acids are beneficial for joint health, it's also important to maintain a healthy balance between omega-3s and omega-6 fatty acids in the diet. Omega-6 fatty acids, found in vegetable oils, processed foods, and meats, can promote

inflammation when consumed in excess. Aim to reduce your intake of omega-6-rich foods and focus on increasing omega-3-rich foods to achieve a healthier balance.

5. Incorporating Omega-3s into Your Diet: To increase your omega-3 intake, aim to include fatty fish in your diet at least twice a week. You can also incorporate plant-based sources of omega-3s, like flaxseeds and walnuts, into your meals and snacks. Consider using flaxseed oil or walnut oil in salad dressings or adding ground flaxseeds to smoothies, oatmeal, or baked goods.

By including omega-3 fatty acids in your diet from a variety of sources, you can help support joint health and potentially reduce inflammation associated with arthritis. However, it's important to consult with a healthcare professional before making significant changes to your diet or starting any new supplements, especially if you have a medical condition or are taking medications.

Understanding Bone Fractures and the Healing Process

Bone fractures are common injuries that can vary in severity and require proper nutrition to support the healing process. The types of fractures include:

1. Closed Fracture: Also known as a simple fracture, this type of fracture does not break the skin.

2. Open Fracture: Also called a compound fracture, this type of fracture involves a break in the skin, which can lead to a higher risk of infection.

3. Stress Fracture: This type of fracture is caused by repetitive stress or overuse and is common in athletes or those who engage in repetitive activities.

4. Comminuted Fracture: In this type of fracture, the bone breaks into several pieces.

5. Compression Fracture: Often seen in the spine, this fracture occurs when the bone collapses due to pressure, such as in osteoporosis.

6. Avulsion Fracture: This type of fracture occurs when a fragment of bone is pulled away by a tendon or ligament.

The bone healing process typically involves several stages:

1. Inflammatory Phase: This initial phase begins immediately after the fracture occurs and can last for several days. Blood clotting occurs at the site of the fracture, and immune cells are recruited to the area to begin the repair process.

2. Reparative Phase: During this phase, which can last for several weeks, new bone tissue begins to form at the fracture site. The bone starts to knit together, and a soft callus forms around the fracture.

3. Remodeling Phase: In the final phase of bone healing, which can last for months to years, the bone remodels and reshapes itself to regain its original strength and structure.

Nutrition plays a crucial role in supporting the bone healing process. Adequate intake of nutrients such as protein, calcium, vitamin D, vitamin C, and other vitamins and minerals is essential for bone health and fracture healing. Protein is necessary for the formation of new bone tissue, while calcium, vitamin D, and other nutrients are vital for bone mineralization and strength. Vitamin C is important for collagen synthesis, which is crucial for the formation of new bone tissue.

Foods to Support Healing During Bone Fracture Recovery

During the recovery process from a bone fracture, nutrition plays a critical role in supporting healing and overall bone health. Consuming a well-balanced diet that includes nutrient-rich foods can provide the essential vitamins, minerals, and other nutrients needed for optimal bone healing. Here are some key foods to include in your diet to support bone fracture recovery:

1. Protein-Rich Foods: Protein is essential for the repair and rebuilding of damaged tissues, including bones. Include lean sources of protein such as poultry, fish, lean meats, eggs, dairy products, legumes, and tofu in your meals to support the healing process.

2. Calcium-Rich Foods: Calcium is a vital mineral for bone health and plays a crucial role in bone mineralization. Include dairy products like milk, yogurt, and cheese, as well as fortified plant-based alternatives, to ensure an adequate intake of calcium during bone fracture recovery.

3. Vitamin D Sources: Vitamin D is necessary for calcium absorption and bone mineralization. Exposure to sunlight is the primary source of vitamin D, but you can also obtain it from fortified foods like milk, orange juice, and cereals, as well as fatty fish such as salmon, mackerel, and tuna.

4. Vitamin C-Rich Foods: Vitamin C is essential for collagen synthesis, which is important for the formation of new bone tissue. Include citrus fruits,

strawberries, kiwi, bell peppers, broccoli, and tomatoes in your diet to boost your vitamin C intake.

5. Vitamin K-Rich Foods: Vitamin K is involved in bone mineralization and helps maintain bone density. Incorporate leafy green vegetables like kale, spinach, Swiss chard, and broccoli, as well as other sources like soybeans and canola oil, to ensure an adequate intake of vitamin K.

6. Magnesium Sources: Magnesium is important for bone formation and mineralization. Include magnesium-rich foods such as nuts, seeds, whole grains, legumes, leafy green vegetables, and fish in your diet to support bone health.

7. Zinc and Copper-Rich Foods: Zinc and copper are trace minerals that play roles in bone formation and tissue repair. Include foods like lean meats, seafood, nuts, seeds, whole grains, and legumes to ensure adequate intake of these minerals.

8. Omega-3 Fatty Acids: Omega-3 fatty acids have anti-inflammatory properties that can help reduce

BONE HEALTH DIET

inflammation and support the healing process. Include fatty fish like salmon, mackerel, and sardines, as well as flaxseeds, chia seeds, and walnuts, in your diet for a good source of omega-3s.

9. Antioxidant-Rich Foods: Antioxidants can help reduce inflammation and oxidative stress, which are important for the healing process. Include a variety of colorful fruits and vegetables, as well as nuts, seeds, and whole grains, to ensure an adequate intake of antioxidants.

10. Hydration: Staying hydrated is essential for overall health and healing. Drink plenty of water throughout the day to support the healing process and maintain optimal hydration.

BONE HEALTH DIET

Chapter 7: Diet for Paget's Disease and Other Bone Disorders

Overview of Paget's Disease: Causes, Symptoms, and Treatment Options

Paget's disease of bone, also known as osteitis deformans, is a chronic bone disorder characterized by abnormal bone remodeling, leading to weakened, enlarged, and misshapen bones. This condition can affect one or multiple bones in the body and often progresses slowly over time. Here's an overview of the causes, symptoms, and treatment options for Paget's disease:

1. Causes: The exact cause of Paget's disease is not fully understood, but it is thought to be related to a combination of genetic and environmental factors. Some research suggests that viral infections, particularly by the paramyxovirus, may trigger the abnormal bone remodeling process seen in Paget's disease.

2. Symptoms: Paget's disease can be asymptomatic in some cases, but it can also cause a range of symptoms, including bone pain, joint pain, warmth over affected bones, bone deformities, fractures, and hearing loss (if the skull is affected). Additionally, overactive bone remodeling can lead to complications

such as osteoarthritis, nerve compression, and an increased risk of bone cancer.

3. Diagnosis: Diagnosis of Paget's disease is typically based on a combination of clinical symptoms, imaging studies (such as X-rays, bone scans, and CT scans), and blood tests to assess bone turnover markers and rule out other conditions with similar symptoms.

4. Treatment: The goal of treatment for Paget's disease is to reduce bone pain, prevent complications, and normalize bone turnover. Treatment options may include:

  - Medications: Bisphosphonates are the primary medications used to treat Paget's disease. They work by inhibiting bone resorption and reducing excessive bone turnover. Other medications, such as calcitonin and pain relievers, may also be prescribed to manage symptoms.

  - Physical Therapy: Physical therapy and regular exercise can help improve joint mobility, muscle strength, and overall function, which can be beneficial for individuals with Paget's disease.

- Surgery: In severe cases or when complications arise, surgery may be necessary to stabilize fractures, correct bone deformities, or relieve nerve compression.

5. Nutrition and Lifestyle Considerations: While there is no specific diet that can cure Paget's disease, maintaining a balanced diet rich in calcium, vitamin D, and other essential nutrients is important for overall bone health. Adequate calcium and vitamin D intake can help support bone strength and minimize the risk of fractures. Additionally, avoiding excessive alcohol consumption and smoking can also benefit bone health.

6. Monitoring and Follow-Up: Regular monitoring of bone health through imaging studies and blood tests is important for individuals with Paget's disease. This can help assess the response to treatment and detect any potential complications early on.

Nutritional Considerations for Managing Paget's Disease and Other Bone Disorders

When managing Paget's disease and other bone disorders, nutrition plays a crucial role in supporting bone health and managing symptoms. Certain dietary modifications can help optimize bone health and minimize the impact of these conditions. Here are some key nutritional considerations for managing Paget's disease and other bone disorders:

1. Calcium and Vitamin D Intake: Adequate calcium and vitamin D intake is essential for maintaining bone health. Calcium-rich foods include dairy products like milk, yogurt, and cheese, as well as fortified plant-based alternatives. Vitamin D can be obtained from exposure to sunlight and from fortified foods such as milk, orange juice, and cereals, as well as fatty fish like salmon and mackerel.

2. Protein Consumption: Protein is essential for bone formation and repair. Include lean sources of protein such as poultry, fish, lean meats, eggs, dairy products, legumes, and tofu in your diet to support bone health.

3. Limiting Alcohol and Caffeine: Excessive alcohol consumption can interfere with bone metabolism and increase the risk of fractures. Limit alcohol intake and avoid excessive caffeine consumption, as caffeine can interfere with calcium absorption.

4. Balanced Diet: A well-balanced diet that includes a variety of fruits, vegetables, whole grains, lean proteins, and healthy fats provides essential nutrients for overall health and bone support.

5. Omega-3 Fatty Acids: Omega-3 fatty acids have anti-inflammatory properties that can benefit individuals with bone disorders by reducing inflammation. Include sources of omega-3s such as fatty fish (salmon, mackerel, sardines), flaxseeds, chia seeds, and walnuts in your diet.

6. Hydration: Staying hydrated is important for overall health, including bone health. Drink plenty of water throughout the day to maintain optimal hydration.

BONE HEALTH DIET

7. Supplements: In some cases, your healthcare provider may recommend calcium, vitamin D, or other supplements to help meet your nutritional needs. Follow your healthcare provider's recommendations regarding supplementation.

8. Consultation with a Registered Dietitian: If you have Paget's disease or another bone disorder, consider consulting with a registered dietitian who can provide personalized dietary recommendations based on your specific needs and medical history.

Bone Health Supplements for Paget's Disease and Other Bone Disorders

For individuals with Paget's disease and other bone disorders, maintaining optimal bone health is crucial for managing symptoms and preventing complications. In addition to a balanced diet, certain supplements may play a role in supporting bone health and addressing specific nutritional needs. Here's a look at some supplements that may be beneficial for individuals with Paget's disease and other bone disorders:

1. Calcium and Vitamin D: Adequate calcium and vitamin D intake is essential for bone health, as these nutrients are crucial for bone mineralization and strength. Many individuals with Paget's disease may require higher levels of calcium and vitamin D supplementation to support bone health. Calcium supplements are available in various forms, such as calcium carbonate and calcium citrate, and should be taken with meals for optimal absorption. Vitamin D supplements, especially vitamin D3 (cholecalciferol), can help ensure adequate levels of this vitamin, which is important for calcium absorption and bone metabolism.

2. Bisphosphonates: Bisphosphonates are a class of medications often used to treat Paget's disease by slowing down bone breakdown and reducing the risk of complications. While bisphosphonates are primarily prescribed as medications rather than dietary supplements, they are an important part of the treatment plan for many individuals with Paget's disease.

3. Magnesium: Magnesium is involved in bone formation and mineralization, and adequate magnesium intake may support bone health. Some research suggests that magnesium supplementation may benefit individuals with certain bone disorders, although more studies are needed to confirm its specific role in Paget's disease.

4. Vitamin K: Vitamin K is important for bone health as it helps regulate calcium and promotes bone mineralization. Some studies have suggested that vitamin K supplementation may improve bone density and reduce fracture risk, particularly in individuals with osteoporosis. Vitamin K2 (menaquinone) is the form of vitamin K most often associated with bone health.

5. Trace Minerals: Trace minerals like zinc, copper, and manganese play important roles in bone health and may be included in bone health supplements. These minerals are involved in bone formation and remodeling processes and may support overall bone health when included as part of a balanced supplement regimen.

BONE HEALTH DIET

6. Omega-3 Fatty Acids: Omega-3 fatty acids have anti-inflammatory properties that may benefit individuals with Paget's disease and other bone disorders by reducing inflammation and supporting overall bone health. Omega-3 supplements are available in various forms, such as fish oil capsules or algae-based supplements.

Chapter 8: Lifestyle Factors

for Bone Health

Exercise and Bone Health:

Importance of Weight-Bearing

Exercises and Resistance Training

Physical activity is crucial for maintaining strong and healthy bones, and certain types of exercise can be particularly beneficial for bone health. Here's why weight-bearing exercises and resistance training are important for promoting bone health:

Weight-Bearing Exercises:

Weight-bearing exercises are physical activities that require your body to work against gravity while standing upright. These exercises are beneficial for bone health because they stimulate the bones to become stronger and denser. Here's an expanded look at the importance and examples of weight-bearing exercises:

1. Importance for Bone Health: Weight-bearing exercises are crucial for maintaining bone density and strength, which is essential for overall bone health. As you engage in these activities, your bones are subjected to the force of gravity, which triggers the bone-forming cells (osteoblasts) to build new bone tissue. Over time, this process helps to maintain or even increase bone density, reducing the risk of osteoporosis and fractures.

2. Types of Weight-Bearing Exercises:
   - High-Impact Exercises: These activities involve repetitive impact or pounding on the bones, which can be particularly effective for improving bone

density. Examples include jogging, running, jumping rope, and high-impact aerobics.

- Low-Impact Exercises: While not as intense as high-impact exercises, low-impact activities still provide the benefits of weight-bearing exercise without the same level of stress on the joints. Examples include walking, elliptical training, stair climbing, and low-impact aerobics.

- Sports and Activities: Many sports and recreational activities naturally involve weight-bearing elements, such as basketball, soccer, tennis, and dancing. These activities can be enjoyable ways to incorporate weight-bearing exercise into your routine.

- Resistance Training: While not strictly weight-bearing in the traditional sense, resistance training with weights or resistance bands can also stimulate bone growth by placing stress on the bones. Exercises like squats, lunges, and leg presses can be particularly effective for targeting the lower body bones.

3. Safety Considerations: When engaging in weight-bearing exercises, it's important to consider your current fitness level, any existing health conditions, and the potential impact on your joints. Start slowly

and gradually increase the intensity and duration of your workouts to allow your bones and muscles to adapt. Use proper form and technique to reduce the risk of injury, and listen to your body's signals to avoid overexertion.

4. Frequency and Duration: Aim for at least 150 minutes of moderate-intensity aerobic activity or 75 minutes of vigorous-intensity aerobic activity per week, combined with muscle-strengthening activities on two or more days a week. This can help you meet the recommended guidelines for physical activity while supporting your bone health.

2. Resistance Training: Resistance training, also known as strength training or weightlifting, involves using weights or resistance bands to strengthen muscles and bones. This type of exercise can help improve bone density, especially when combined with weight-bearing activities. Resistance training can be done using free weights, weight machines, resistance bands, or even your body weight (e.g., push-ups, squats). It targets specific muscle groups and can help improve

overall strength and balance, which is important for reducing the risk of falls and fractures.

3. Impact and Loading: Weight-bearing exercises and resistance training provide mechanical stress to the bones, which is necessary for bone remodeling and adaptation. The impact and loading placed on the bones during these activities help stimulate the bone-forming cells (osteoblasts) to build new bone tissue, leading to stronger and denser bones.

4. Bone Density Maintenance: Regular weight-bearing exercises and resistance training can help maintain bone density and reduce the risk of osteoporosis, a condition characterized by weak and brittle bones. By engaging in these types of exercises, you can help preserve bone mass and reduce the likelihood of fractures as you age.

5. Safety Considerations: It's important to perform weight-bearing exercises and resistance training safely to minimize the risk of injury. Start with light weights or resistance and gradually increase the intensity as your strength improves. Always use proper form and

technique to avoid strain or injury to your muscles and bones. If you have any existing health conditions or concerns, consult with a healthcare provider or a certified fitness professional before starting a new exercise program.

Alcohol Consumption and Bone Health

Alcohol consumption can have both positive and negative effects on bone health, depending on the amount consumed and individual factors. Here's a look at the impact of alcohol on bone health and guidelines for moderation:

1. Effect of Alcohol on Bone Density: Chronic heavy alcohol consumption is associated with an increased risk of osteoporosis and bone fractures. Excessive alcohol intake can interfere with the body's ability to absorb calcium and other essential nutrients for bone health, leading to decreased bone density and strength.

2. Moderate Alcohol Consumption: While heavy alcohol consumption can harm bone health, moderate

alcohol intake may not have the same negative effects and could potentially offer some benefits. Moderate alcohol consumption is generally defined as up to one drink per day for women and up to two drinks per day for men. One drink is equivalent to 12 ounces of beer, 5 ounces of wine, or 1.5 ounces of distilled spirits.

3. Potential Benefits of Moderate Alcohol Intake: Some studies suggest that moderate alcohol consumption, particularly in the form of red wine, may have protective effects on bone health. Red wine contains polyphenols, such as resveratrol, which have been shown to have potential bone-protective properties. However, the evidence is not conclusive, and more research is needed to fully understand the relationship between moderate alcohol consumption and bone health.

4. Risks of Excessive Alcohol Consumption: Excessive alcohol intake can negatively impact bone health in several ways. It can interfere with the body's ability to absorb calcium, decrease bone formation, and increase the risk of falls and fractures due to impaired coordination and balance. Chronic heavy alcohol

consumption is also associated with an increased risk of developing osteoporosis and other bone-related conditions.

5. Balancing Alcohol Consumption and Bone Health: If you choose to consume alcohol, it's important to do so in moderation and be mindful of its potential impact on bone health. Consider limiting your alcohol intake to within the recommended guidelines and balancing it with a diet rich in calcium, vitamin D, and other nutrients important for bone health. Additionally, engaging in regular weight-bearing exercise and maintaining a healthy lifestyle can help support bone health and minimize the potential negative effects of alcohol on bones.

6. Consulting a Healthcare Professional: If you have concerns about how alcohol consumption may be affecting your bone health, or if you have a history of heavy alcohol consumption, it's important to discuss this with a healthcare professional. They can provide personalized recommendations based on your individual health status and help you make informed

BONE HEALTH DIET

decisions about alcohol consumption and its impact on your bone health.

Smoking and Bone Health

Smoking has detrimental effects on bone health, impacting bone density and the body's ability to heal from injuries, fractures, and other bone-related conditions. Here's a closer look at how smoking affects bone health:

1. Reduced Bone Density: Smoking is associated with lower bone density, which increases the risk of osteoporosis and fractures. Nicotine and other harmful chemicals in tobacco smoke can interfere with the production and function of osteoblasts, the cells responsible for bone formation. As a result, smokers may experience accelerated bone loss, particularly in the hips and spine.

2. Delayed Fracture Healing: Smoking can delay the healing process for fractures and other bone injuries. Nicotine and carbon monoxide in tobacco smoke can impair blood flow to the bones, slowing down the

delivery of essential nutrients and oxygen needed for healing. This delay in the healing process can prolong recovery time and increase the risk of complications.

3. Increased Risk of Osteoporosis: Smoking is a significant risk factor for osteoporosis, a condition characterized by weak and brittle bones. Chronic smoking can lead to a decrease in bone mass and quality, making the bones more susceptible to fractures and injuries.

4. Impact on Bone Healing after Surgery: For individuals undergoing orthopedic surgeries or procedures involving bone, smoking can negatively impact the outcome. Smoking can impair the body's ability to form new bone tissue and repair damaged bones, leading to longer recovery times and an increased risk of complications such as non-union (failure of bones to heal) or delayed union (slow healing of bones).

5. Secondhand Smoke Exposure: In addition to the direct effects of smoking, exposure to secondhand smoke can also impact bone health, especially in

children and adolescents whose bones are still developing. Secondhand smoke exposure has been linked to reduced bone density and an increased risk of fractures in children.

6. Reversing the Effects: Quitting smoking can help mitigate the negative effects on bone health. Studies have shown that individuals who quit smoking may experience improvements in bone density and a reduced risk of fractures over time. However, it's important to note that the benefits of quitting smoking may take time to become apparent, and the earlier smoking cessation occurs, the better the chances of preserving bone health.

Chapter 9: Bone Health

Across the Lifespan

Childhood and Adolescence:

Nutritional Needs for Bone

Development

Childhood and adolescence are critical periods for bone development, as bones grow and reach peak bone mass during these stages. Proper nutrition plays a crucial role in supporting optimal bone growth and mineralization during this time. Here's a look at the nutritional needs for bone development in growing children and teens, along with the recommended daily amounts:

1. Calcium: Calcium is essential for building strong bones and teeth. Growing children and teens require varying amounts of calcium based on their age:
    - Children aged 1-3 years: 700 mg/day
    - Children aged 4-8 years: 1,000 mg/day
    - Children aged 9-18 years: 1,300 mg/day

Good sources of calcium include dairy products like milk, yogurt, and cheese, as well as fortified plant-based alternatives like almond milk or soy milk. Other sources include leafy green vegetables, tofu, and calcium-fortified foods.

2. Vitamin D: Vitamin D is necessary for calcium absorption and bone mineralization. The recommended daily intake of vitamin D for children and teens is:
    - Children aged 1-18 years: 600 IU/day

Vitamin D can be obtained through sunlight exposure as well as from dietary sources such as fatty fish (e.g., salmon, mackerel), egg yolks, and fortified foods like cereals and orange juice.

3. Protein: Protein is essential for the formation and growth of bones and muscles. The recommended daily intake of protein for children and teens is based on their age and gender:
   - Children aged 4-8 years: 19 grams/day
   - Boys aged 9-13 years: 34 grams/day
   - Girls aged 9-13 years: 34 grams/day
   - Boys aged 14-18 years: 52 grams/day
   - Girls aged 14-18 years: 46 grams/day

Good sources of protein include lean meats, poultry, fish, eggs, dairy products, legumes, nuts, and seeds.

4. Vitamin K, Magnesium, and Phosphorus: These nutrients are also important for bone health. While specific daily recommendations vary by age and gender, including a variety of foods rich in these nutrients as part of a balanced diet can contribute to overall bone health.

BONE HEALTH DIET

Pregnancy and Breastfeeding: Importance of Calcium and Vitamin D

During pregnancy and breastfeeding, adequate nutrition is crucial for both the mother's health and the development of the baby. Calcium and vitamin D play particularly important roles in supporting bone health during these phases of life.

1. Calcium: Calcium is essential for the development of the baby's bones and teeth. During pregnancy, the growing fetus relies on the mother's calcium supply to build its own skeletal system. If the mother's calcium intake is insufficient, the fetus may draw calcium from the mother's bones, potentially increasing the risk of bone density loss for the mother. Additionally, adequate calcium intake during pregnancy can reduce the risk of pregnancy-induced hypertension and pre-eclampsia.

2. Vitamin D: Vitamin D is necessary for the absorption of calcium and the proper mineralization of bones. During pregnancy and breastfeeding, vitamin D is essential for the development of the baby's bones and

teeth. Adequate vitamin D levels in the mother are also important for her own bone health. Vitamin D deficiency during pregnancy has been linked to an increased risk of pre-eclampsia, gestational diabetes, and low birth weight.

3. Sources of Calcium and Vitamin D: Good dietary sources of calcium include dairy products such as milk, yogurt, and cheese, as well as fortified foods like tofu, orange juice, and cereals. Green leafy vegetables, almonds, and sesame seeds are also sources of calcium. Vitamin D can be obtained from sunlight exposure and certain foods such as fatty fish (e.g., salmon, mackerel), egg yolks, and fortified foods like milk and cereals. In some cases, healthcare providers may recommend vitamin D supplements during pregnancy and breastfeeding to ensure adequate intake.

4. Supplementation: Pregnant and breastfeeding women should discuss their calcium and vitamin D needs with their healthcare providers. Depending on individual circumstances and dietary habits, supplementation may be recommended to ensure

sufficient intake of these nutrients. Prenatal vitamins often contain calcium and vitamin D, but additional supplements may be advised based on blood test results and other factors.

5. Breastfeeding: Breast milk is a good source of calcium and vitamin D for the baby. However, the mother's own intake of these nutrients remains important to support her own bone health while breastfeeding. It's important for breastfeeding mothers to continue consuming calcium-rich foods and maintaining adequate vitamin D levels.

Aging and Bone Health: Dietary Considerations for Older Adults

As individuals age, maintaining bone health becomes increasingly important to prevent the risk of osteoporosis and fractures. Dietary considerations play a crucial role in supporting bone health in older adults. Here are some key dietary factors to consider:

1. Calcium and Vitamin D: Calcium and vitamin D are essential nutrients for bone health. Calcium is

necessary for bone structure and strength, while vitamin D is essential for calcium absorption. Older adults should ensure adequate intake of both nutrients to support bone health. Good sources of calcium include dairy products, leafy green vegetables, fortified foods, and supplements if necessary. Vitamin D can be obtained from sunlight exposure and fortified foods such as milk, orange juice, and cereals, as well as supplements.

2. Protein: Protein is important for maintaining muscle mass and bone strength. Older adults should include sources of lean protein in their diet, such as poultry, fish, beans, lentils, and tofu. Adequate protein intake can help support muscle and bone health, reducing the risk of falls and fractures.

3. Fruits and Vegetables: Fruits and vegetables are rich in vitamins, minerals, and antioxidants that support overall health, including bone health. They provide essential nutrients like vitamin C, which is important for collagen formation, and vitamin K, which plays a role in bone mineralization. Older adults should aim to

BONE HEALTH DIET

include a variety of colorful fruits and vegetables in their diet to ensure they get a wide range of nutrients.

4. Omega-3 Fatty Acids: Omega-3 fatty acids have anti-inflammatory properties and may help reduce the risk of osteoporosis and fractures. Sources of omega-3s include fatty fish (such as salmon, mackerel, and sardines), flaxseeds, chia seeds, and walnuts. Including these foods in the diet can provide benefits for both bone and overall health.

5. Hydration: Staying hydrated is important for overall health and can benefit bone health as well. Older adults should aim to drink an adequate amount of fluids, primarily water, throughout the day to maintain hydration and support bone health.

6. Limiting Alcohol and Caffeine: Excessive alcohol consumption and caffeine intake can have negative effects on bone health. Older adults should moderate their alcohol intake and limit caffeine consumption to support bone health.

BONE HEALTH DIET

7. Medical Conditions and Medications: Some medical conditions and medications can affect bone health. Older adults should work with their healthcare provider to manage any conditions or medications that may impact bone health, such as osteoporosis medications, corticosteroids, or other medications that affect bone density.

Chapter 10: Creating a Personalized Bone Health Plan.

Assessing Your Bone Health: Tools for Evaluating Bone Density and Overall Bone Health

Evaluating your bone health is an important step in creating a personalized plan to maintain or improve bone density and overall bone health. Several tools and assessments can help you and your healthcare provider assess your bone health status. Here are some common tools used for evaluating bone health:

1. Bone Density Testing (DXA Scan): Dual-energy X-ray absorptiometry (DXA or DEXA) is the most widely used method for measuring bone mineral density (BMD). It is a painless and non-invasive procedure that uses low-dose X-rays to measure the mineral content of bones, usually in the hip and spine. The results are reported as T-scores and Z-scores, which compare your bone density to that of a healthy young adult (T-score) or someone of your age, sex, and ethnicity (Z-score).

2. Fracture Risk Assessment Tools: Fracture risk assessment tools, such as the FRAX® tool, estimate the 10-year probability of a major osteoporotic fracture (including hip, spine, forearm, or shoulder fractures) or hip fracture based on various risk factors, including age, sex, weight, height, previous fractures,

family history, smoking status, alcohol intake, and the presence of other medical conditions.

3. Biochemical Markers of Bone Turnover: Blood and urine tests can measure biochemical markers of bone turnover, which reflect the rate at which bone is being broken down and rebuilt. These markers can provide insight into bone health and bone metabolism, although they are not typically used as standalone diagnostic tools for osteoporosis.

4. Clinical Assessment: A comprehensive clinical assessment by a healthcare provider includes a review of your medical history, physical examination, evaluation of risk factors for osteoporosis and fractures, and discussions about lifestyle factors that can impact bone health, such as diet, exercise, and medications.

5. Imaging Studies: In addition to DXA scans, other imaging studies such as quantitative computed tomography (QCT) or peripheral DXA (pDXA) scans may be used to assess bone density in specific areas

of the body or to monitor changes in bone density over time.

6. Genetic Testing: In some cases, genetic testing may be used to assess the risk of developing certain bone disorders or conditions that affect bone health.

Developing a Balanced Diet for Bone Health

A balanced diet plays a crucial role in supporting bone health by providing essential nutrients that contribute to bone strength and density. Here are some tips for creating a diet plan that supports bone health:

1. Calcium-Rich Foods: Calcium is a key nutrient for bone health, so it's important to include calcium-rich foods in your diet. Good sources of calcium include dairy products like milk, yogurt, and cheese, as well as fortified plant-based alternatives like soy milk and almond milk. Leafy green vegetables, such as kale, collard greens, and broccoli, also contain calcium.

2. Vitamin D Sources: Vitamin D is essential for calcium absorption and bone health. Include foods that are naturally rich in vitamin D, such as fatty fish (salmon, mackerel, and tuna), egg yolks, and fortified foods like milk, orange juice, and cereals. Sunlight exposure is also an important source of vitamin D.

3. Protein: Protein is important for bone health as it provides the building blocks for bone tissue. Include

lean sources of protein in your diet, such as poultry, fish, lean meats, eggs, dairy products, legumes, and tofu.

4. Fruits and Vegetables: Fruits and vegetables are rich in vitamins, minerals, and antioxidants that support overall health, including bone health. Aim to include a variety of colorful fruits and vegetables in your diet to ensure you get a wide range of nutrients.

5. Whole Grains: Whole grains like brown rice, quinoa, oats, and whole wheat bread provide important nutrients like magnesium and phosphorus, which are essential for bone health. They also contribute to overall dietary balance and provide sustained energy.

6. Healthy Fats: Omega-3 fatty acids found in fatty fish, flaxseeds, chia seeds, and walnuts have anti-inflammatory properties that may benefit bone health by reducing inflammation. Include these sources of healthy fats in your diet.

7. Limit Sodium and Caffeine: High sodium intake can lead to calcium loss in the urine, which can weaken

BONE HEALTH DIET

bones over time. Limit your intake of processed foods, which are often high in sodium. Additionally, excessive caffeine consumption can interfere with calcium absorption, so it's best to moderate your intake of caffeinated beverages.

8. Stay Hydrated: Proper hydration is important for overall health, including bone health. Drink plenty of water throughout the day to stay hydrated.

9. Alcohol in Moderation: Excessive alcohol consumption can interfere with the body's ability to absorb calcium and may affect bone density. If you choose to drink alcohol, do so in moderation.

10. Consult a Registered Dietitian: If you have specific dietary concerns or health conditions that may impact your bone health, consider consulting a registered dietitian who can help you create a personalized diet plan that meets your nutritional needs and supports bone health.

Long-Term Maintenance: Strategies for Maintaining Bone Health Throughout Life

BONE HEALTH DIET

Maintaining optimal bone health is a lifelong commitment that requires ongoing attention and care. As you age, your bone health needs may change, and it's important to adjust your lifestyle and habits accordingly. Here are some strategies for long-term maintenance of bone health:

1. Nutrition: Continue to prioritize a balanced diet rich in calcium, vitamin D, protein, and other essential nutrients for bone health. As you age, your body's ability to absorb certain nutrients may change, so it's important to ensure that your diet provides adequate nutrition to support bone health.

2. Regular Physical Activity: Engage in regular weight-bearing and muscle-strengthening exercises to maintain bone density and strength. Weight-bearing exercises include activities like walking, jogging, dancing, and hiking, which help stimulate bone growth and maintain bone mass. Strength-training exercises, such as lifting weights or using resistance bands, can help strengthen muscles and bones.

BONE HEALTH DIET

3. Fall Prevention: Preventing falls is crucial for maintaining bone health, especially as you age. Take steps to minimize fall risks in your home and surroundings, such as removing tripping hazards, installing handrails and grab bars, and ensuring adequate lighting.

4. Healthy Lifestyle Choices: Avoid smoking and limit alcohol consumption, as both can negatively impact bone health. Smoking can decrease bone density, while excessive alcohol intake can interfere with calcium absorption and increase the risk of fractures.

5. Regular Bone Health Assessments: Schedule regular check-ups with your healthcare provider to assess your bone health and discuss any changes in your lifestyle, medications, or health status that may impact your bone health.

6. Medication Adherence (If Applicable): If you are taking medications to support bone health, such as osteoporosis medications, ensure that you take them as prescribed and follow your healthcare provider's recommendations for monitoring and management.

BONE HEALTH DIET

7. Bone Health Education: Stay informed about bone health and osteoporosis prevention by staying up-to-date with the latest research and recommendations. Consider joining support groups or educational programs focused on bone health to learn from others and stay motivated.

8. Regular Health Screenings: Maintain regular health screenings, including bone density tests (DXA scans), to monitor your bone health and detect any changes or issues early on.